NEW OLD FRIENDS

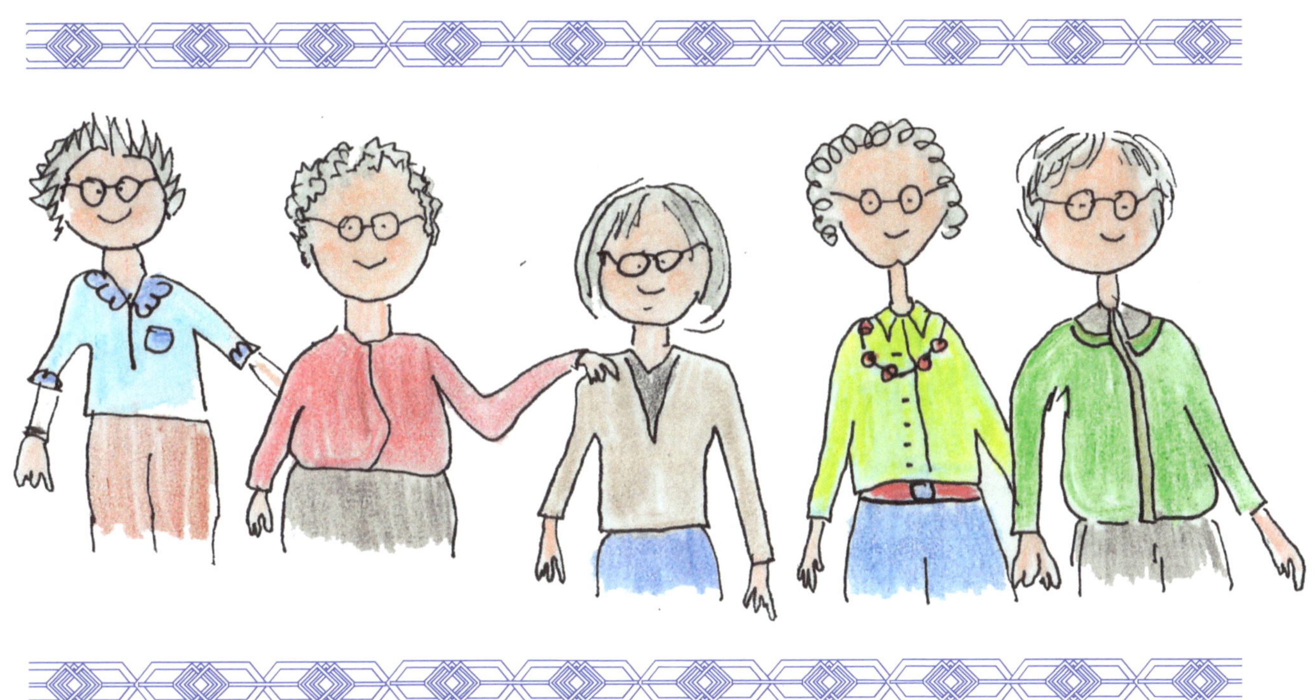

HEADING TOWARD 100

WRITTEN & ILLUSTRATED BY

ANNA COHN DONNELLY

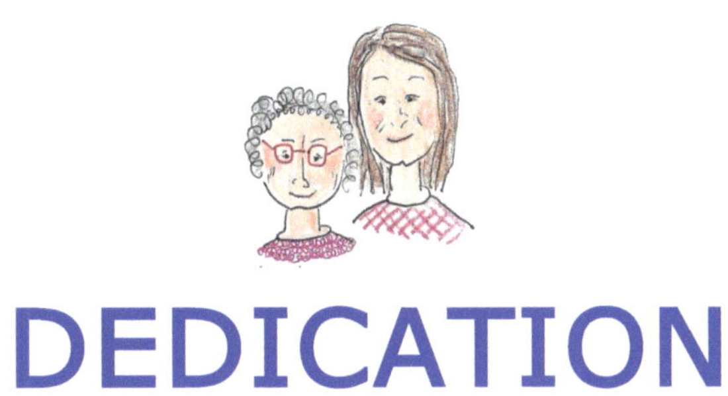

DEDICATION

I dedicate this book to Mimi, my mom.

It is said that parents are their children's first and most important teacher. Mimi, you have been and continue to this day to be mine! You are my role model for how to be a good person. You are kind, thoughtful, nonjudgmental, and also pragmatic. You have no meanness in your body, no anger, no resentment, no jealousies. You make goodness accessible to people who know you. You offer unconditional love to all your children and grandchildren and you offer the same to all your friends.

You showed us how to live what we, your children, call "the French Fry Principle": equal shares for all.

With love!

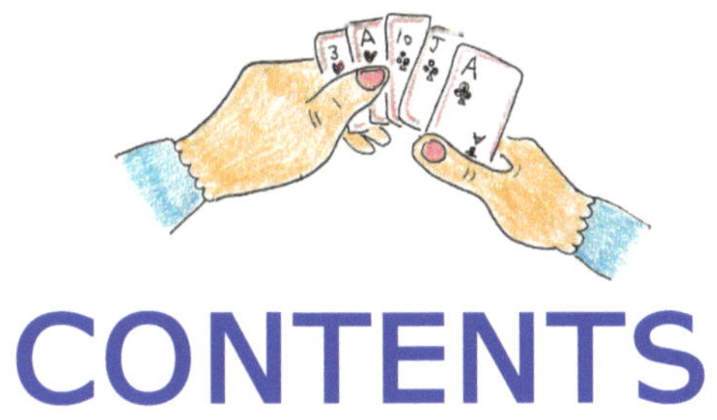

CONTENTS

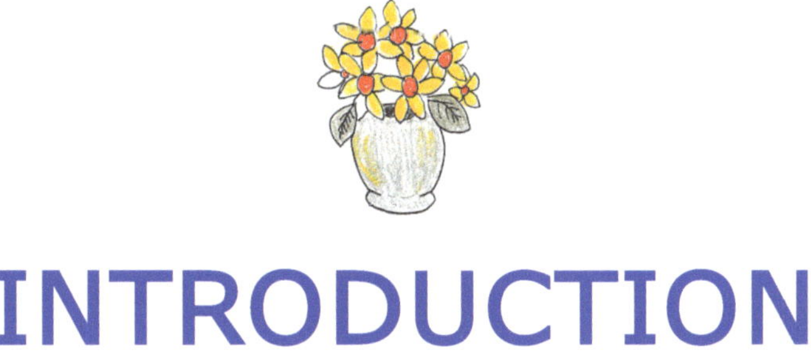

INTRODUCTION

This book is about a special group of women in their late 80s and 90s who can see 100 on the horizon, including my mom, Mimi. I was motivated to write this book having had informal conversations with Mimi's friends over the last decade or so and finding myself constantly inspired by them—their positive outlook and joy of living.

I wanted to better understand them, the lives they have lived, and their thoughts about aging. So, I conducted interviews with fourteen of them (including Mimi) to learn more about where they have come from and what keeps them going. The following pages contain their thoughts.[1]

All reside in the Residence[2], a senior living community. All have had rich and wonderful lives. All have experienced great sorrow in their long lifetimes.

They have lost their parents, husbands, for some a child or grandchild, siblings, other relatives, and friends. They have given up the homes and neighborhoods where they raised their families. They have lost a lot physically. They know that growing older could become even harder.

But, they are in life to live. They each have a belief in their own capacity to cherish life even as they carry their losses. They understand that attitude is everything. They have mostly positive attitudes. Importantly, as they age they find they actually gain a lot.

1   This symbol ◄♦► which you'll notice throughout, separates comments from different people.
2   A fictional name.

MIMI'S STORY

Mimi moved into the Residence fifteen years ago with her second husband. With this decision, as with all things, she was very pragmatic as she thought about the move, right on down to wanting to maintain her independence by having a place to wash her car. She explains:

> *"I had never thought about where I would live as I got older. And then a friend moved into a senior living community and wrote to me about how terrific it was. I decided to explore this possibility.*

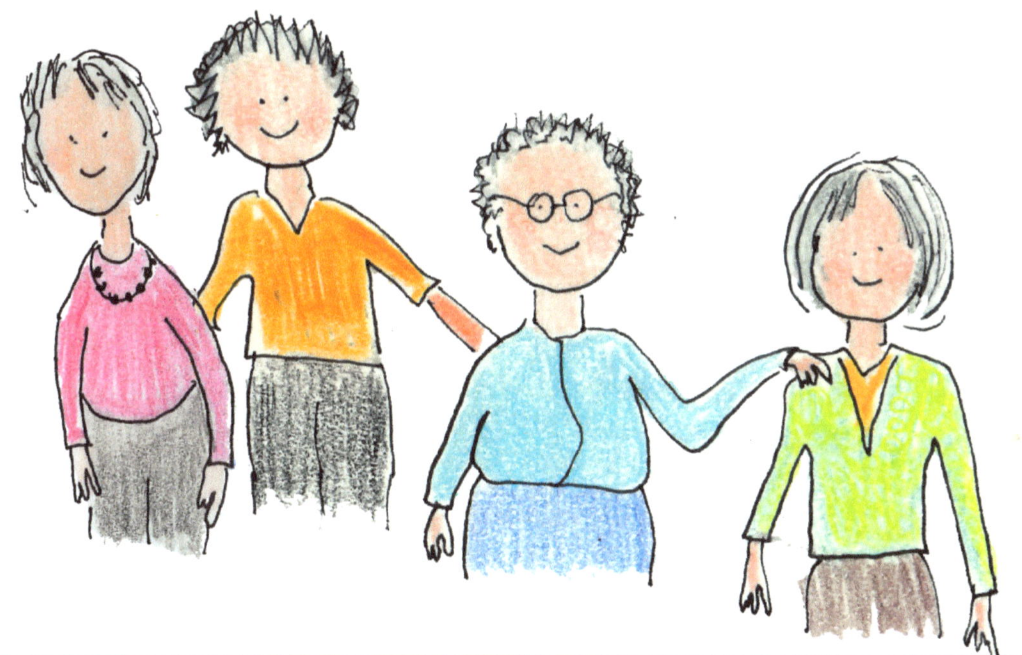

"I wanted to find a place to live with other people my age. I wanted at least one of my five children nearby. I wanted a comfortable place, not a house, but a residence with a spot where I could wash my car.

"My daughter Anna hunted for a place for me. She found the Residence. It was brand new with no waiting list. I could have one of the Villas which came with a two-car garage—plenty of space for car washing. And Anna lived fifteen minutes away.
I decided to move in.

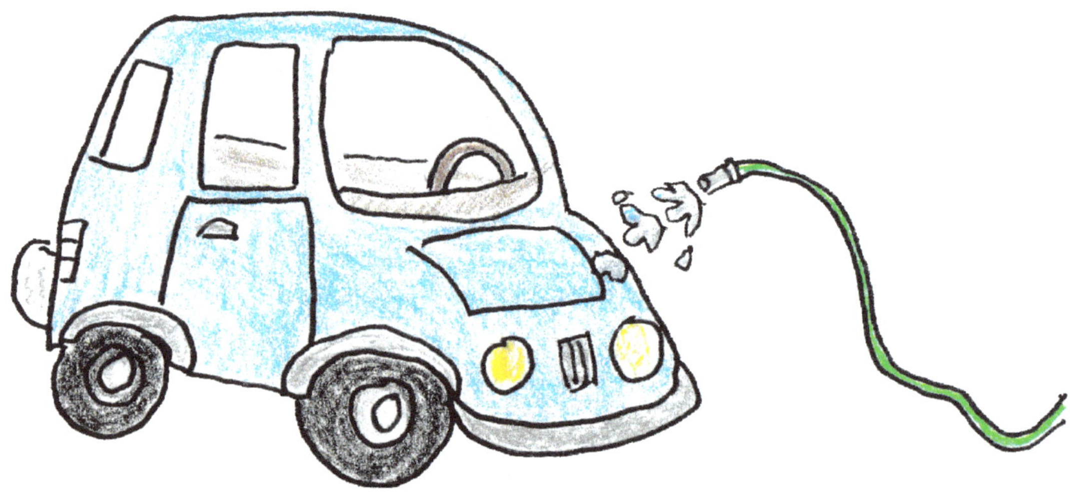

"I have found the Residence to be very comfortable and attractive. It offers all kinds of opportunities to keep healthy: from exercise classes to nutritious meals, lifelong learning activities to arts, and even gardening.

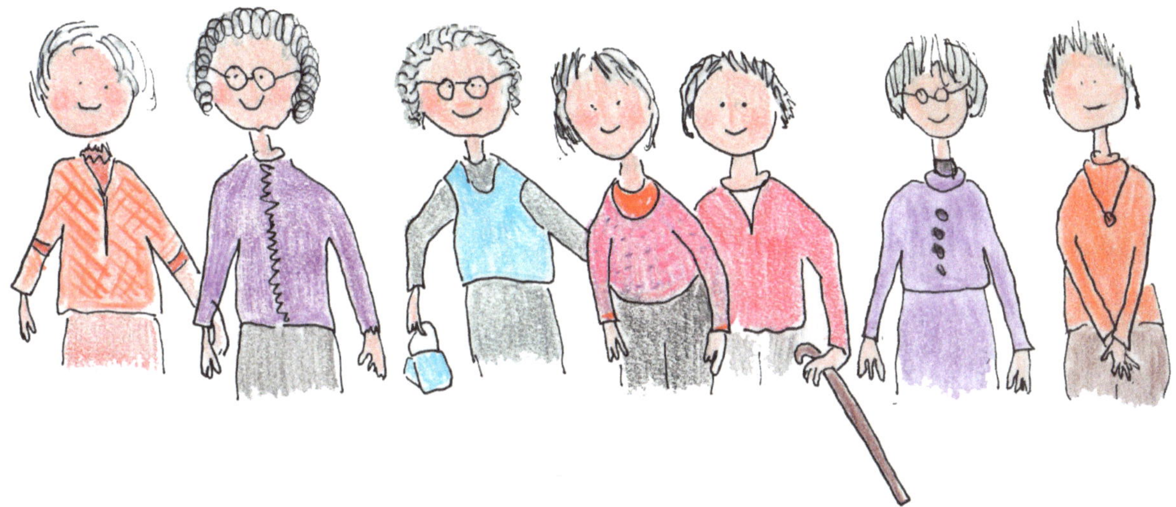

"After a lifetime of feeding a family and caring for a house, I don't have to worry about buying food or cooking and cleaning up. But if I want to cook, the Residence bus will take me to the local grocery store. I don't have to worry about how I will get to a doctor's appointment, the Residence staff will drive me.

"Living here gives me a boost in connecting with others. I've done lots of different activities: ceramics, needlepoint, play reading, flower arranging, bridge. I've made a lot of friends. If I were living in my own house, outside of a community like this, I would not have anywhere near as much contact with other people.

"For someone my age, having just turned 99, I am in good health. I am not stressed or frustrated with my life. And now, as I approach 100, I don't think about

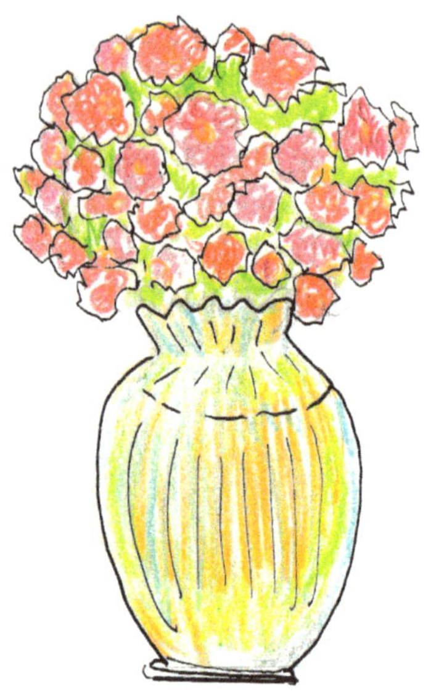

the fact that I am so old in a
negative way. I have a positive
view—I just think about the fact
that I am still alive and lucky
to be this age and to have this
community of people."

New Old Friends

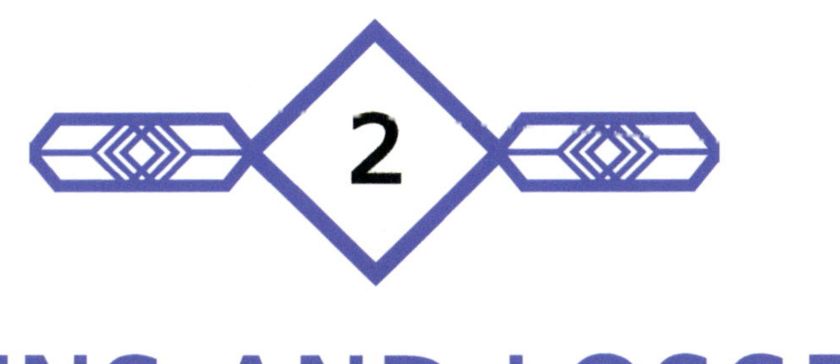

GAINS AND LOSSES

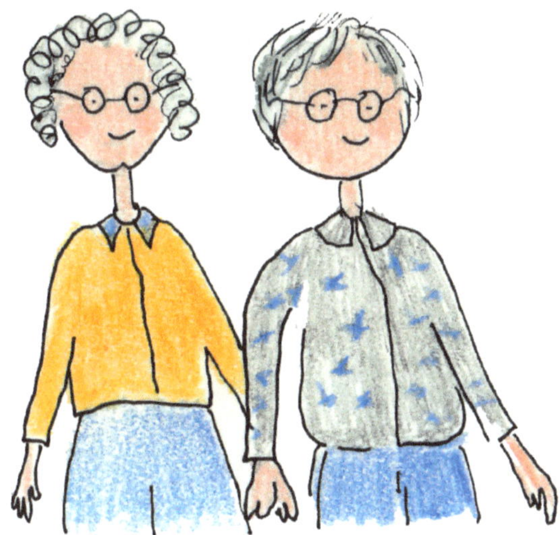

"My friend Nancy passed away last month. It really hurts. Makes me feel lost. She was a really good friend. We were like best friends."

Mimi has just turned 99. And Nancy was 95. They had been friends for close to fifteen years at the Residence, where they met. They had dinner together several a times week, were often bridge partners, stopped by most days to check up on each other, or perhaps to play a game of Scrabble. They cared about each other. They had both lost other close, late-in-life friends during those fifteen years and certainly many other friends and family in their lifetimes.

And it always hurts. As Mimi said:

"People die, but time goes by, so you just keep moving forward. And what do I do with my emotions? There is nothing to do but feel the hurt."

⊲◆⊳

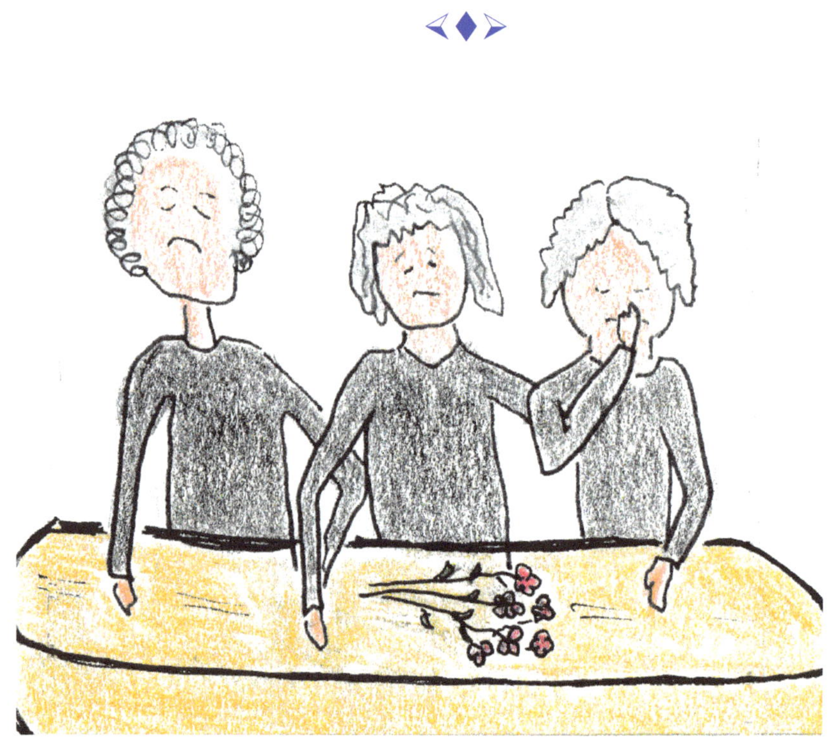

For all, the losses have been deeply painful. For some the losses started too early in life and were unexpected, as a few explain:

"I was 32 years old. I was living on a military base in California with our five young children, ages less than a year to six years old, when I was notified my husband,

a fighter pilot, had been killed. I moved my brood back to Little Rock and raised my children by myself with help from my family."

"My daughter was a single gal working downtown in an office building. One day there was a fire in her building and she did not survive. I have never gotten over the pain of losing her. Others here have lost a child. We share that pain together."

Other losses offered the chance to say good-by:

"I lost my husband twenty years ago. He had been in poor health. Then, my only son died seventeen years ago from cancer at age 54, just one week before I moved into the Residence. He was the one who encouraged me to move here. My two daughters and I were with him during his last few weeks."

"My oldest child had cancer—non-Hodgkin's lymphoma. He had been through all the possible treatments. He was living in Berkeley, California and called me on a Friday, explained that he only had a few days to live, and asked me to come visit as soon as I could. My granddaughter's Bat Mitzvah was on Saturday.

"Early Sunday morning I flew from Chicago to California. I made my way to my son's hospital and found him surrounded by family, friends, and colleagues.

"He asked most of the others to leave the room. And he took my hands and spoke to me:

> *"I am told that the worst pain a person can experience is the loss of a child and I want you to know that I am so very sorry to cause you that pain."*

He died several days later."

<◆>

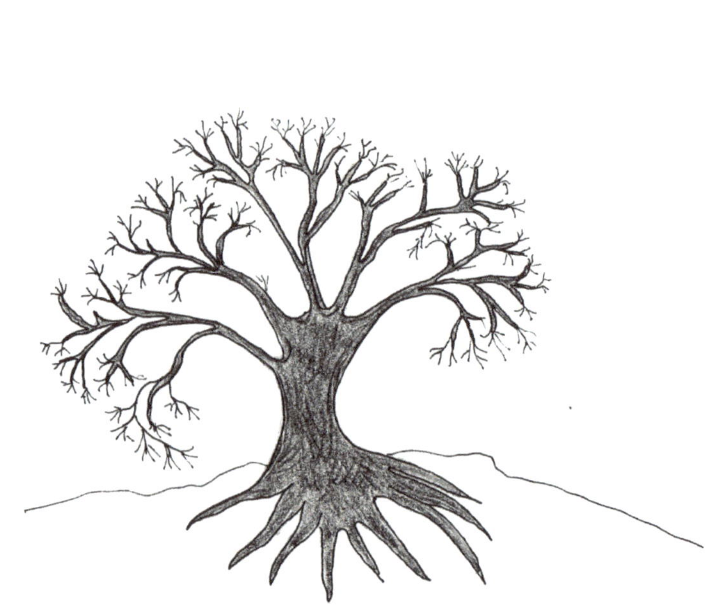

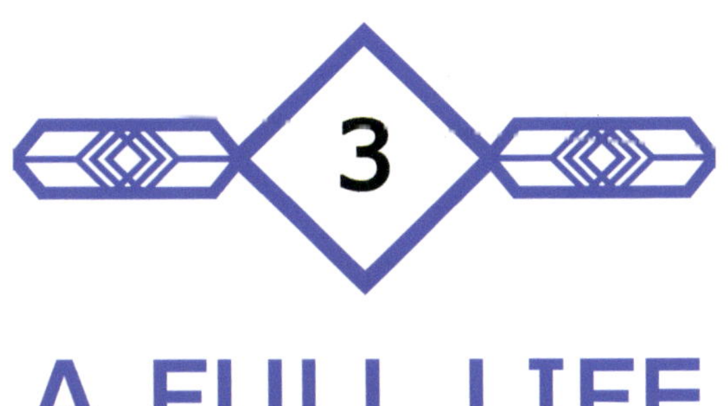

3

A FULL LIFE

These ladies were born in and around the 1920s. They led very active and interesting lives. They are a smart bunch. Several were the valedictorians of their high school classes and one was president of the Student Council.

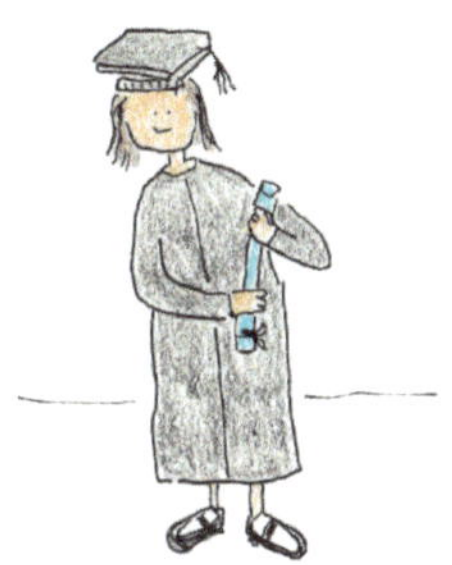

Most attended and finished college. One borrowed $500 from her brother to cover her freshman year costs. Some worked to pay for their education. The parents of others paid their way. Some completed graduate degrees. One won a Fulbright scholarship which took her to Burma.

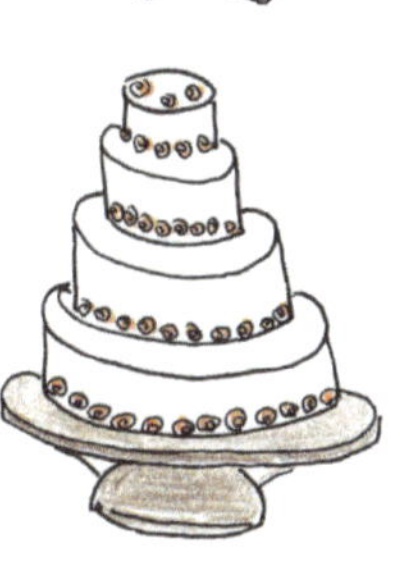

As was true of women born in the early 1920s, they married in their early to mid-twenties, in a number of cases to their high school or even grade school sweethearts. Each had a number of children—two or three or four or five. Time was taken up feeding and caring for their families and their homes. Most worked before marriage: teaching, taking short-hand for an attorney, helping in a dentist's office. Few had careers outside the home once they started their families. One launched a career in marketing and advertising once her children were all in school.

Most volunteered: chair of the local Girl Scouts, founder of a health-related charity, political organizer, part of the church choir, member of a nonprofit board, hospital aide. And they had hobbies: painting, needlepoint, pottery, and bridge.

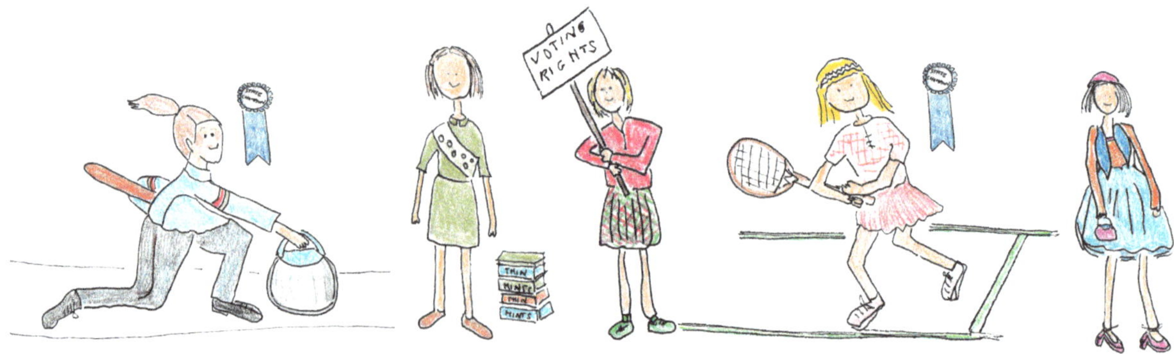

They lived active lives before they married and many continued those activities once married:

> *"I started curling as a school girl and I played well into my adulthood. Our team won the state championship! I was the 'Skip', the person in charge. Curling and being a team member is a metaphor for life. It requires cooperation and appreciation of the other person. And it keeps you stimulated."*

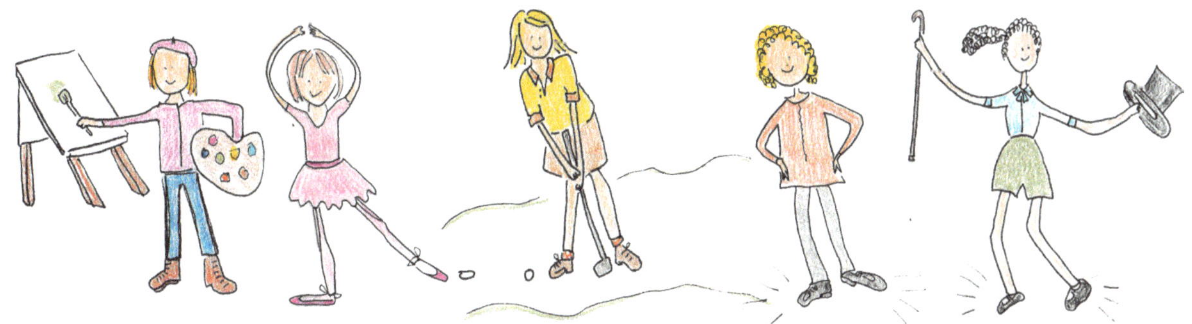

"*I started playing tennis when I was eight years old. In those early days I used a wooden racket. I played most of my life. Won several state championships.*"

"*I was a dancer, a professional tap dancer. We had a group—long after college. We danced at nursing homes and the like. Made money and had a good time. I stopped tap dancing eight years ago.*"

They pursued quite a variety of interests: one was a fashion model, another a ballet dancer, a third a lifelong golfer, and another an avid sailor and cyclist.

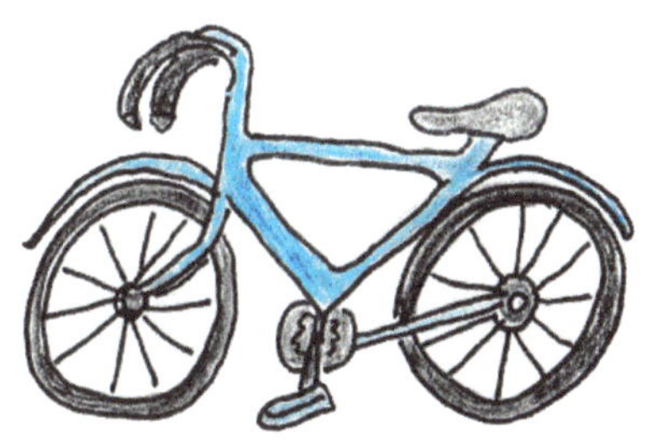

They followed their husbands and moved their families as careers took them across the country and the world—including destinations throughout Europe and Asia.

Each of these women has a keen sense of who she is, using words like independent, loyal, leader, organizer, and helper. Most say they are joiners, easy to get along with, open-minded, happy, friendly. Some say they have lots of pep. Others say energy or not, they are comfortable in their lives and with aging. And they mostly look forward with a positive attitude.

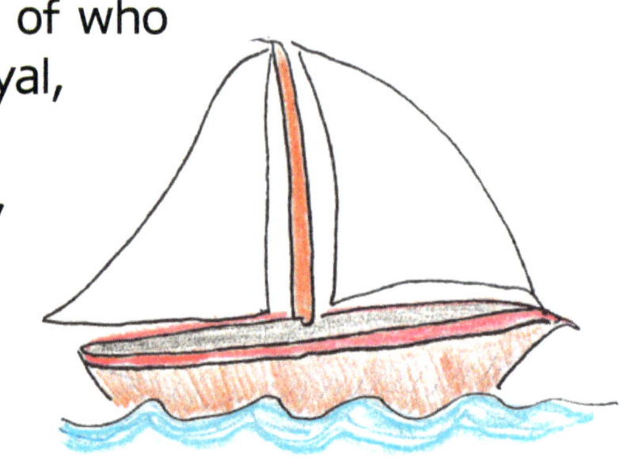

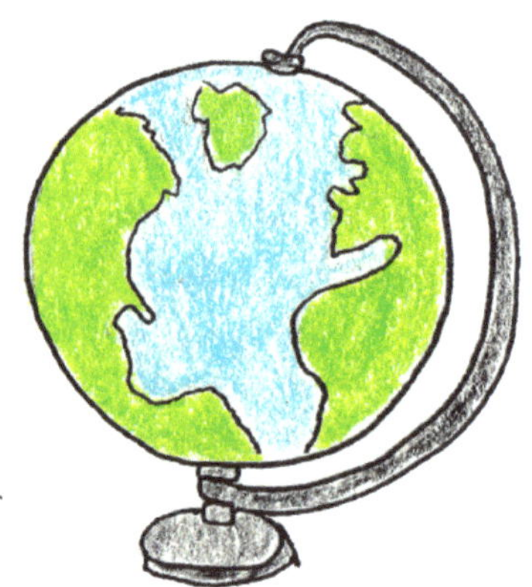

Perhaps the most important description is this:

"I am a family person; my kids, grandkids, and great grandkids are the world to me."

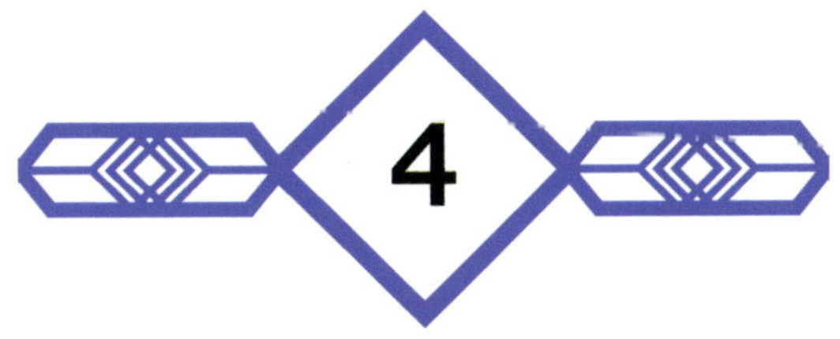

4

A NEW KIND OF HOME

At some point, while in their late seventies and early eighties, each of these women started to think about where she would live as she aged. Each explored the idea of a senior living community and each discovered the Residence.

The Residence is a senior living community with a focus on taking care of the body, mind, and soul. Everything from housekeeping to meal preparation is provided so residents can take advantage of all the community has to offer.

The Residence Wellness Center is staffed seven days a week by a licensed nurse. Medical professionals, including audiologists and podiatrists, visit the Center regularly. The Residence

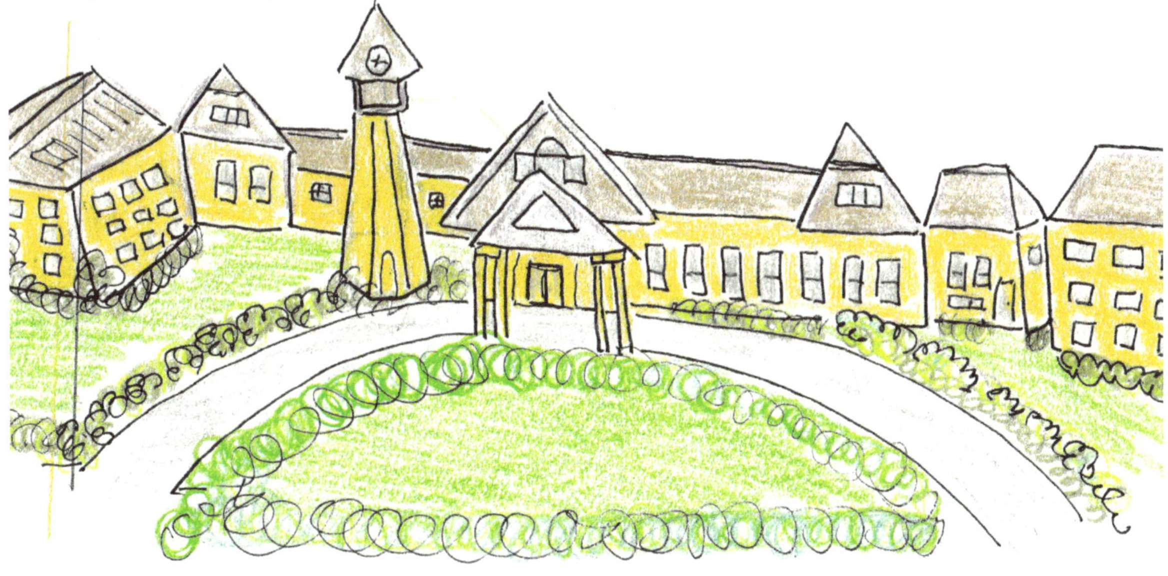

provides residents with a continuum of care on site including assisted living, skilled nursing, and memory support services.

There is an onsite library fully stocked with current magazines, best-selling books, daily local and national newspapers, books on tape, and a computer room with weekly tech assistance.

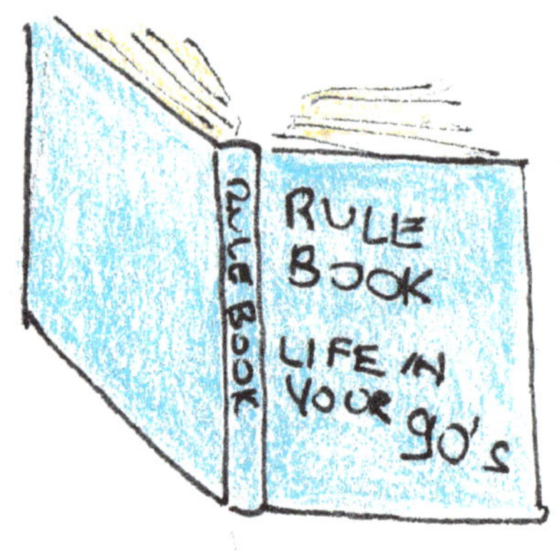

A fitness center has a full array of work-out equipment, an indoor pool, many types of exercise classes, and personal training. There is a beauty salon. Just outside is a large grass putting green and ample land set aside for gardening: vegetables, herbs, and flowers.

Some of the many activities are tai chi, yoga, bridge, Bocce ball, line dancing, choral singing, play reading, book group, computer lab. Classes are offered on a variety of topics including painting, ceramics, chess, acting, and more. Events include trips to theater, symphony concerts, the lyric opera, and the botanic garden.

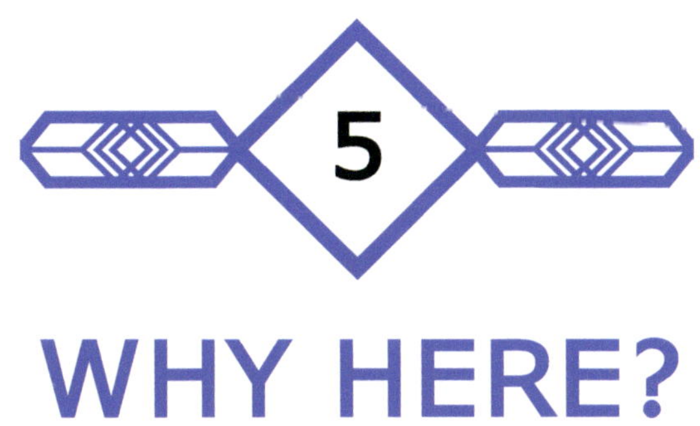

5

WHY HERE?

Why did they come to the Residence? Here is what several had to say:

"I wanted independence, to take care of myself, but to be near one of my children. And, the Residence was new ... I thought it would be fun to live in a new community."

⊰ ♦ ⊱

"The moment we came to visit I knew it was for me, so open and beautiful, so many activities, and my husband fell in love with the chandelier in the cocktail lounge."

⊰ ♦ ⊱

"I was elated to leave a big house, neither my husband nor I could handle all the upkeep: the raking of leaves, the shoveling of snow."

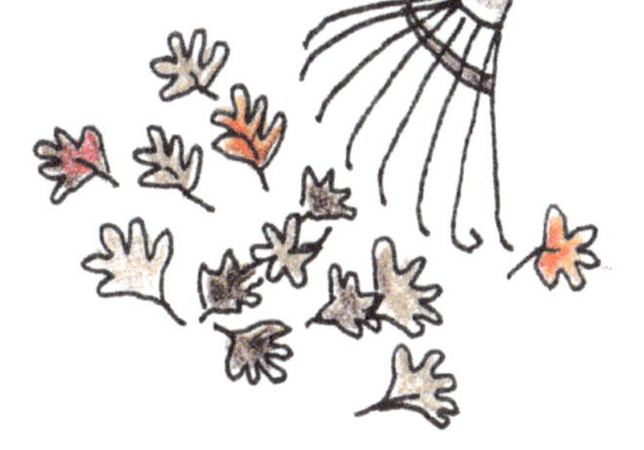
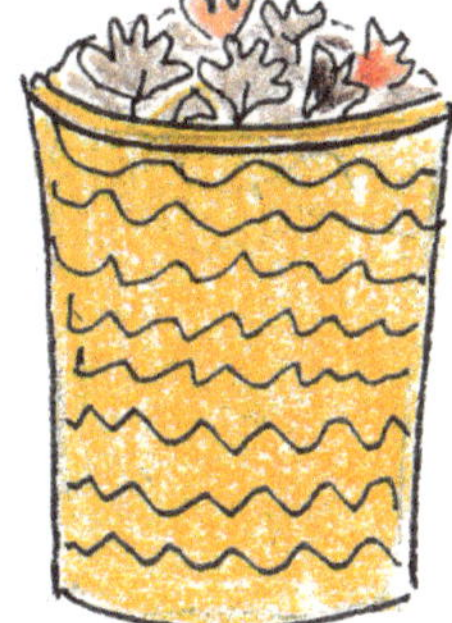

⊰ ♦ ⊱

"We moved in for community, for friends. We realized as we got older we'd be isolated if we stayed in our house."

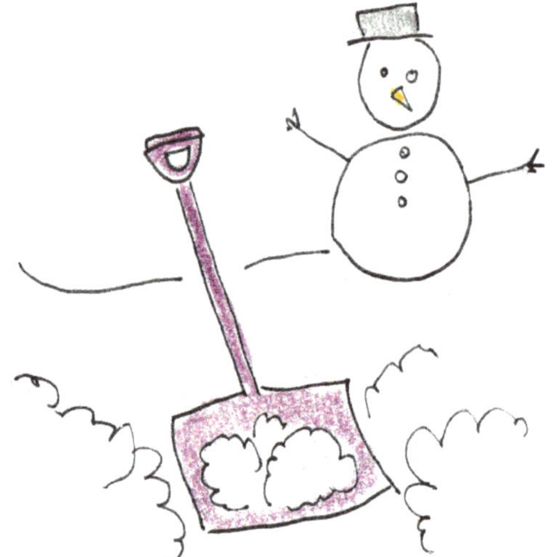

Changing customs in how families dealt with aging certainly influenced some:

"My father and my husband's mother lived with us for seventeen years. Three generations under one roof. They were sweet and interesting. My kids learned a lot from the older

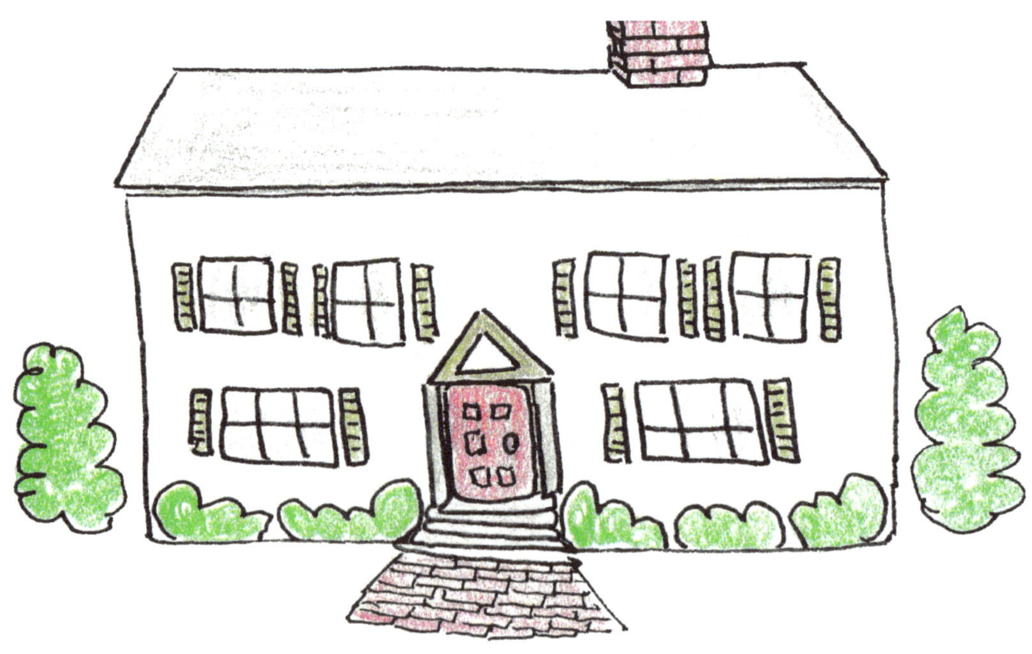

generation. But times have changed. I wanted some independence and wanted my kids to have some too."

And one had this to say:

"I moved to the Residence because I knew it was all downhill and I needed help going downhill."

For most, the move to the Residence meant downsizing, leaving the home where they had raised their family, a home full of possessions:

"Once I decided it was time for me to move, I realized I had a big job ahead of me. Imagine fitting a life-time of stuff into a one-bedroom apartment. Happily my children helped me."

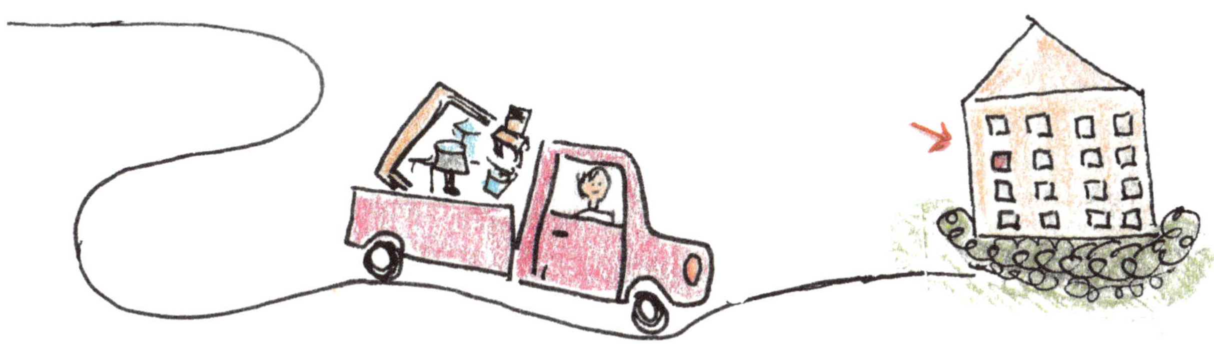

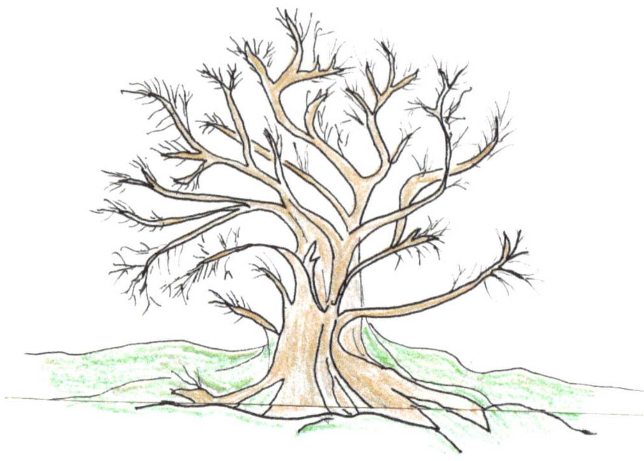

For some it was more than household furnishings that had to be
left behind:

"*Our house was hard to leave. It had a big elm tree.
150 years old. We loved that tree. We hated to leave it
behind.*"

6

BUSY DAYS

There are so many activities one might pursue at the Residence. It is easy to have a full life, but one that, of necessity, changes over time:

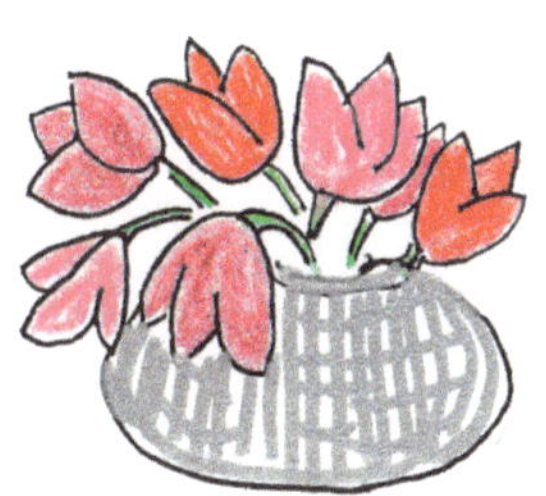

"I started out getting involved in many things. I played bridge, just as I had much of my life. I went to play-reading, often selecting the play we would read or taking on a part. I joined flower-arranging just as it was getting started. Every Friday morning a small group of ladies would meet in the kitchen and arrange fresh flowers in vases for all the tables in the dining rooms. I enjoyed the needlepoint group which met each Monday morning and had lunch together."

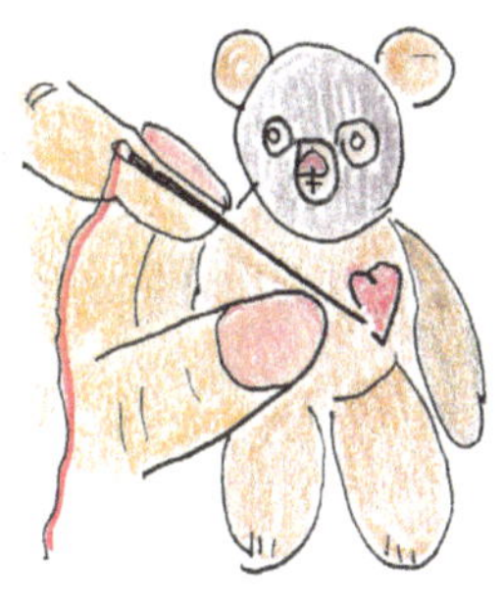

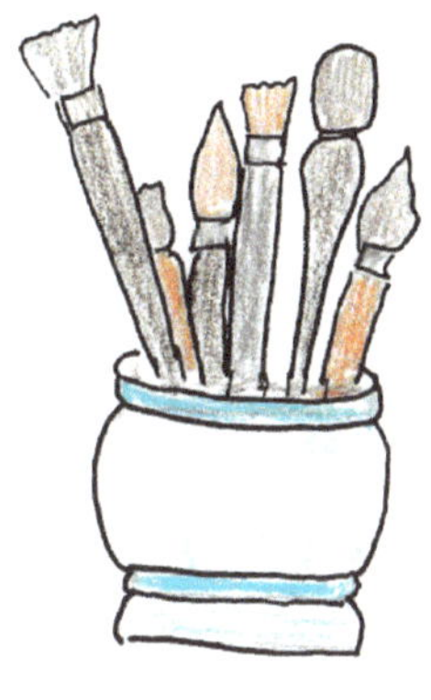

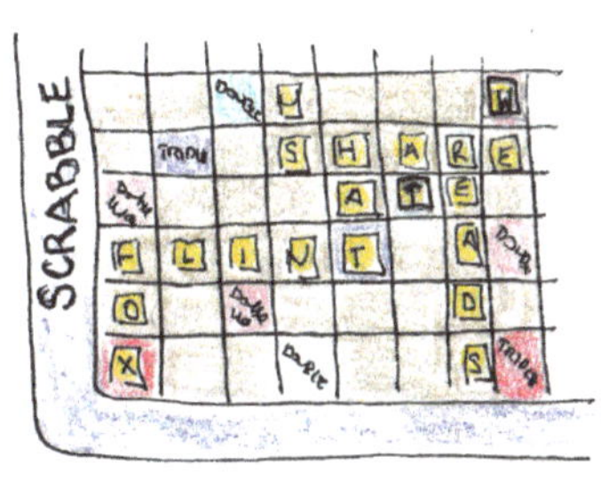

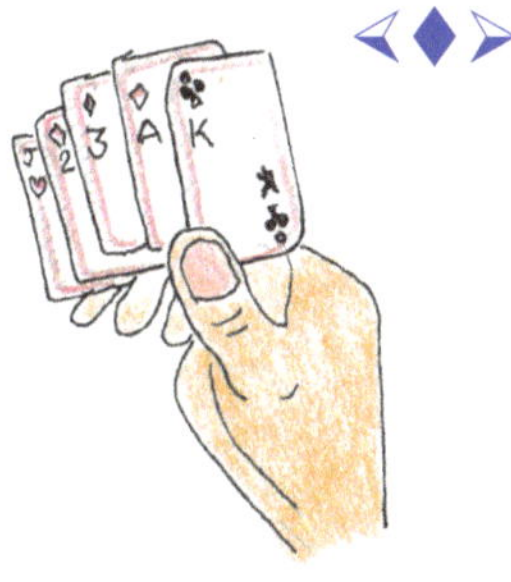

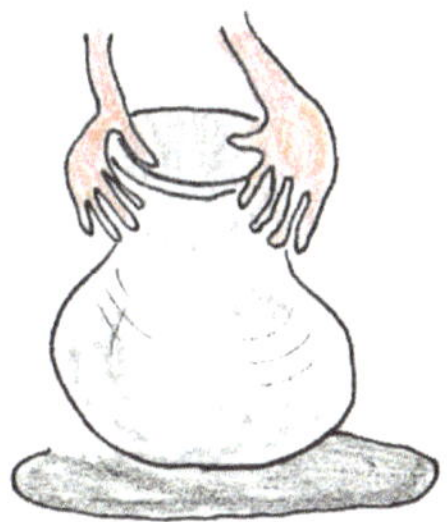

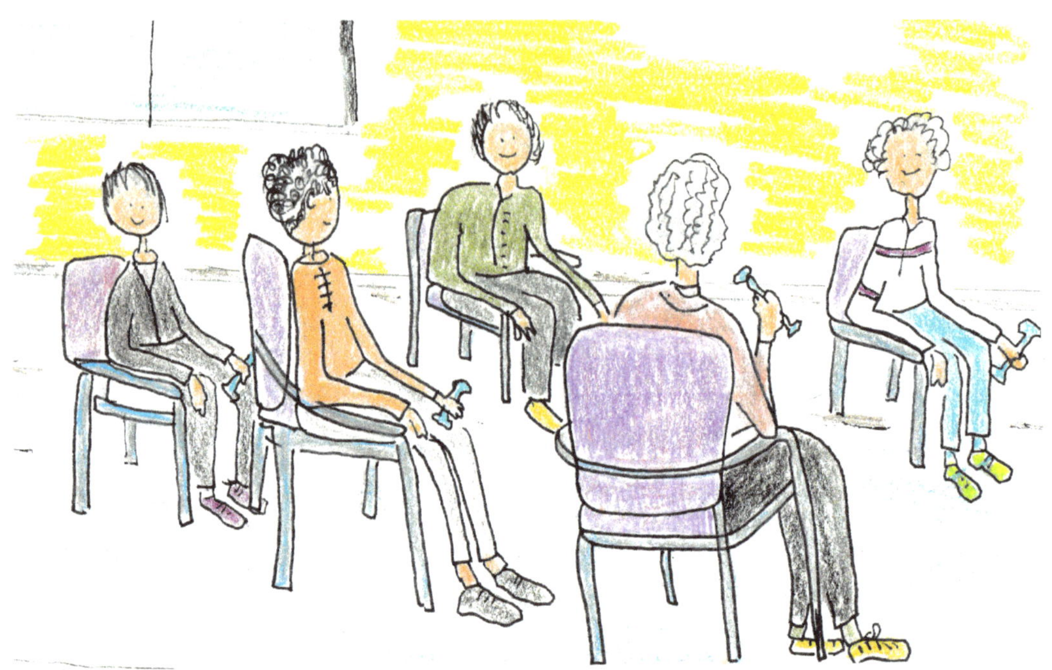

"I tried bocce ball and Strength and Balance. As I got older, the flower arranging became difficult, as did bocce ball. And I replaced Strength and Balance with Sit and Be Fit."

"I used to do everything ... I liked to be busy. I would exercise daily, usually swimming, and play bridge a lot, short story telling, current events, Sit and Be Fit, Strength and Balance, bocce ball, flower arranging. I still

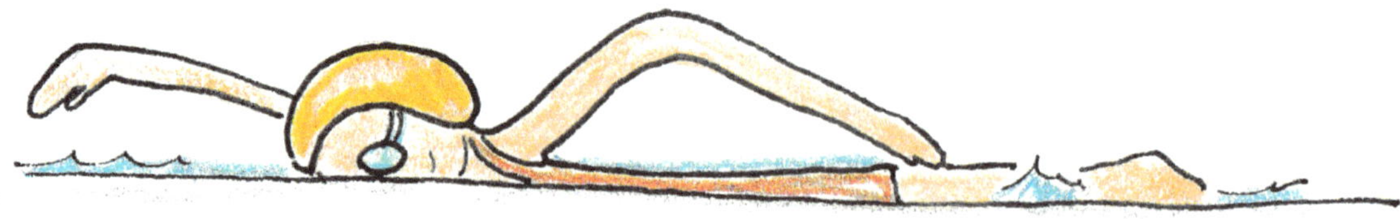

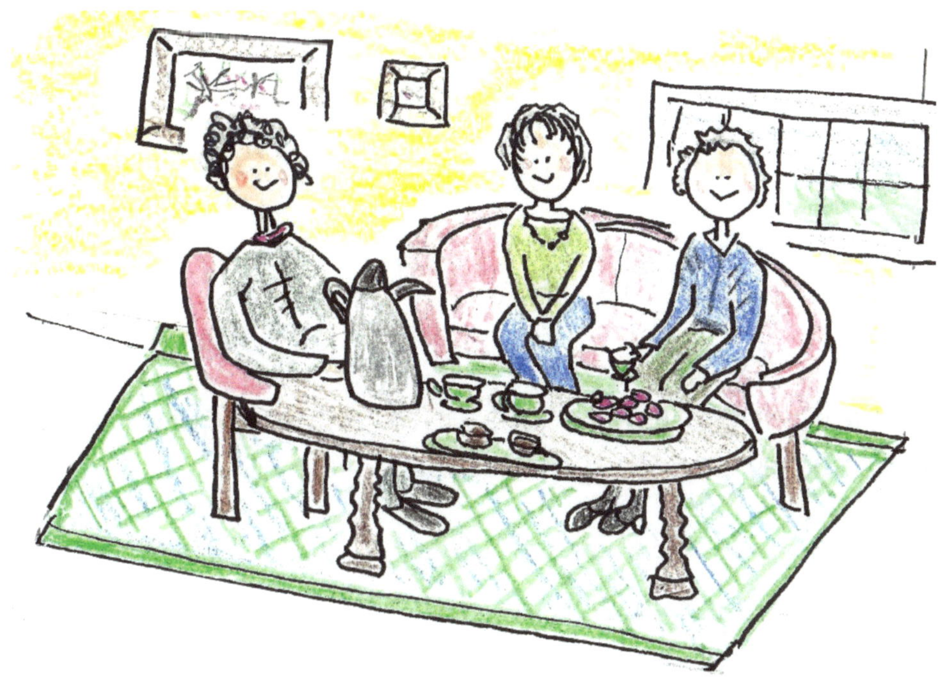

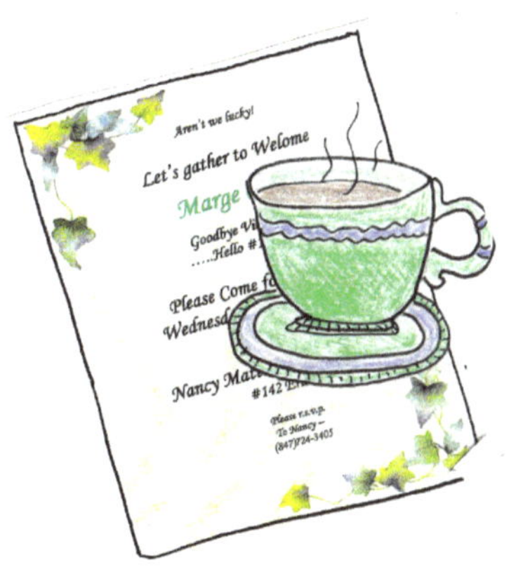

have lots of energy but not quite as much. For a number of years I was head of the Hospitality Committee; we would have a welcome tea for new residents and take them to dinner when they first arrived. Now I just help out a little and I have been pulling back on some of my other activities."

7

STEPS IN AGING

Health and wellbeing are not constants. Aging figures in as explained by some, and changes things.

"Aging comes slowly. First I was a bit unsteady. I got a cane. It took me a while before I started to use it. Then my balance got really bad. The cane didn't work so I got a walker. When my stamina diminished I could have transitioned to a wheel chair. But no, that seemed too old for me. I decided on an electric cart. When I drove down the hallways on it I wanted to yell out 'Watch out everyone, here I come!' I never did hit anybody, just a bunch of walls and some doors. But with no 'Rules of the Road' so to speak, combined with narrow hallways not built to allow two way traffic on electric scooters, at some point I realized it was

time to go back to the walker. When I tire, I can just stop
and sit on it for a few moments."

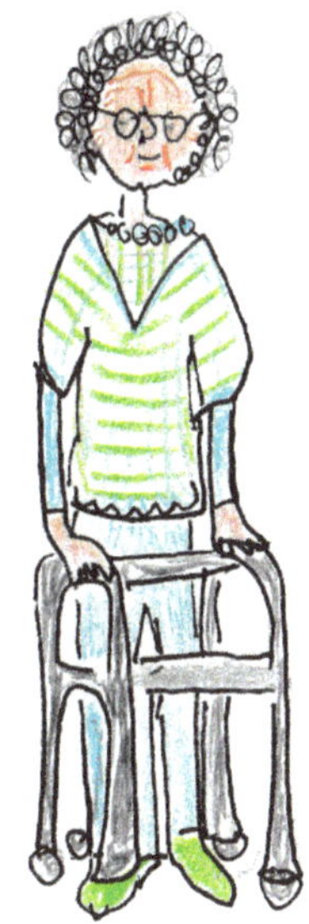

"When I first moved into the Residence
I was proud that I was living
independently. Over time I came to
understand that I needed a bit of
help: in my apartment, with my
clothes and getting breakfast,
and the like. With the help of my
children, I got a part-time caregiver.
As the years went by it became
clear that I really needed someone
with me during the day and into
the evening. So, we arranged for the caregiver
to come for ten hours a day Monday through
Friday and found a second person to come
on the weekends. Turns out I woke up a
lot during the night and needed some help
getting out of bed to go to the bathroom.
What started as very part-time assistance
then turned into 24-hour, seven days a week
care since. I am almost 100. I think that that
is OK."

"I was fine until I fell one morning when I was 94 and
broke my jaw in three places. For close to two months

I had some ladies help with my daily living. I healed faster than the doctors said I would and was back at all my activities soon enough. Then, a year and a half later I fell and broke my hip. I got a hip replacement two days later, spent six weeks at the Residence's Care Center where I had daily physical therapy and then went home. My children lined up 24-hour care for me. Three wonderful women take turns being with me. They are marvelous. They take care of everything for me: making sure I stay active with bridge, needlepoint, ceramics, and they even organize my social calendar."

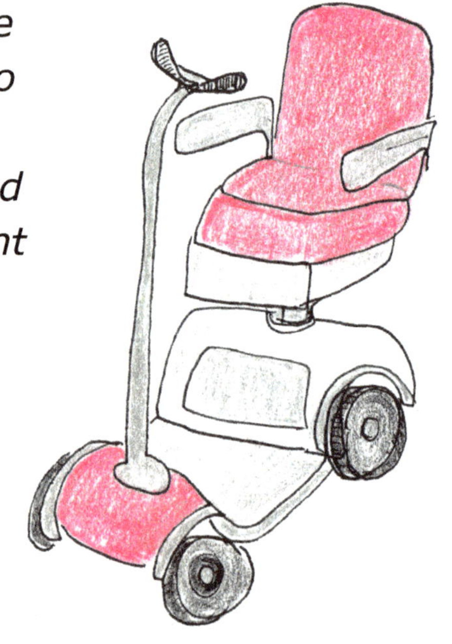

⊰◆⊱

8

CARRYING ON

With great expectations and some hesitation, ten to fifteen years ago these women moved into the Residence. They accepted the notion that this was, as one said, an experiment in growing older. And here's what they think these many years later:

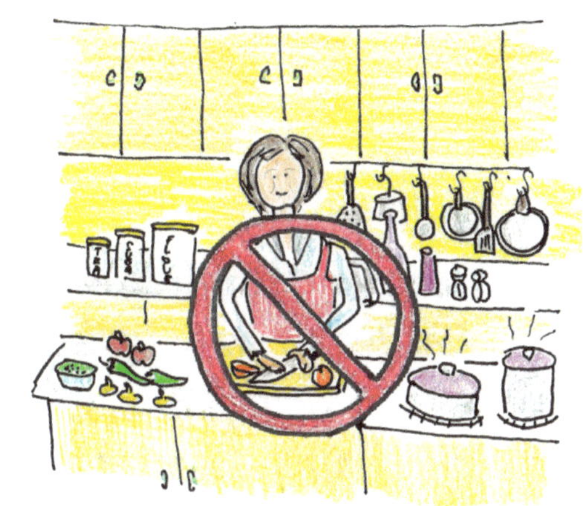

"Life is wonderful here. I have more friends here than ever before—friends who check up on each other and make sure you are okay ... it's a unique kind of friendship—like family."

"Even if you lose your sight or your hearing or you lose your balance there are still lots of things to do."

"I am happy to be here as I get older. I do less stressful things. For example: NO CLEANING and NO COOKING! And if anything goes wrong, even

if it's just a light bulb blowing out, I just call security. Everything is taken care of!"

Life for these ladies is good. But aging brings its challenges:

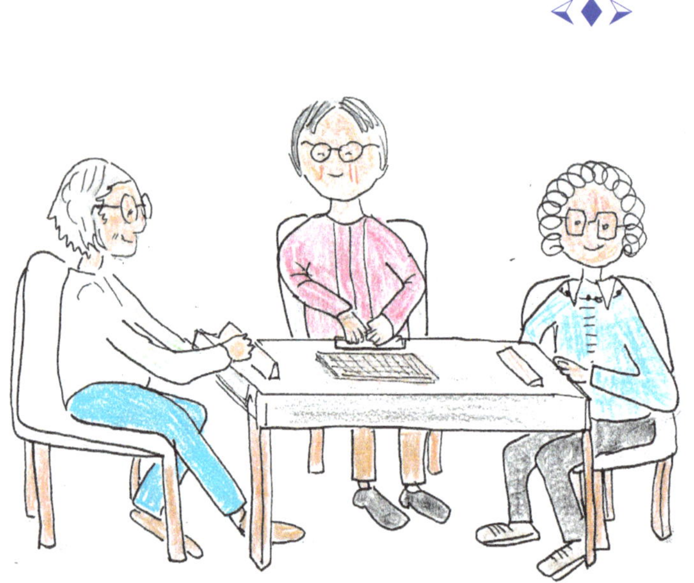

"I don't have as much energy as I used to."

"My health keeps going down."

"As we get older we get limited. It's harder to travel. It's harder to walk up stairs. It is harder to walk. It is harder to get going. Everything is just harder, even eating. Salad gets stuck in my teeth!"

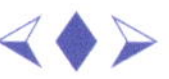

Or, as one observed:

"The very hardest thing is that you make new friends, they become an important part of your life and as we all get older, eventually some will die. Losing these new old friends is very hard!"

So what keeps these women going even as they age? What is their reason to get up each morning?

"Living near one of my children is great. Having my children, grandchildren, and even great grandchildren, come visit, which they do often, is wonderful. But it is the friendships I've made here that keep me going. We check on each other, we support each other, and we accept each other as we age."

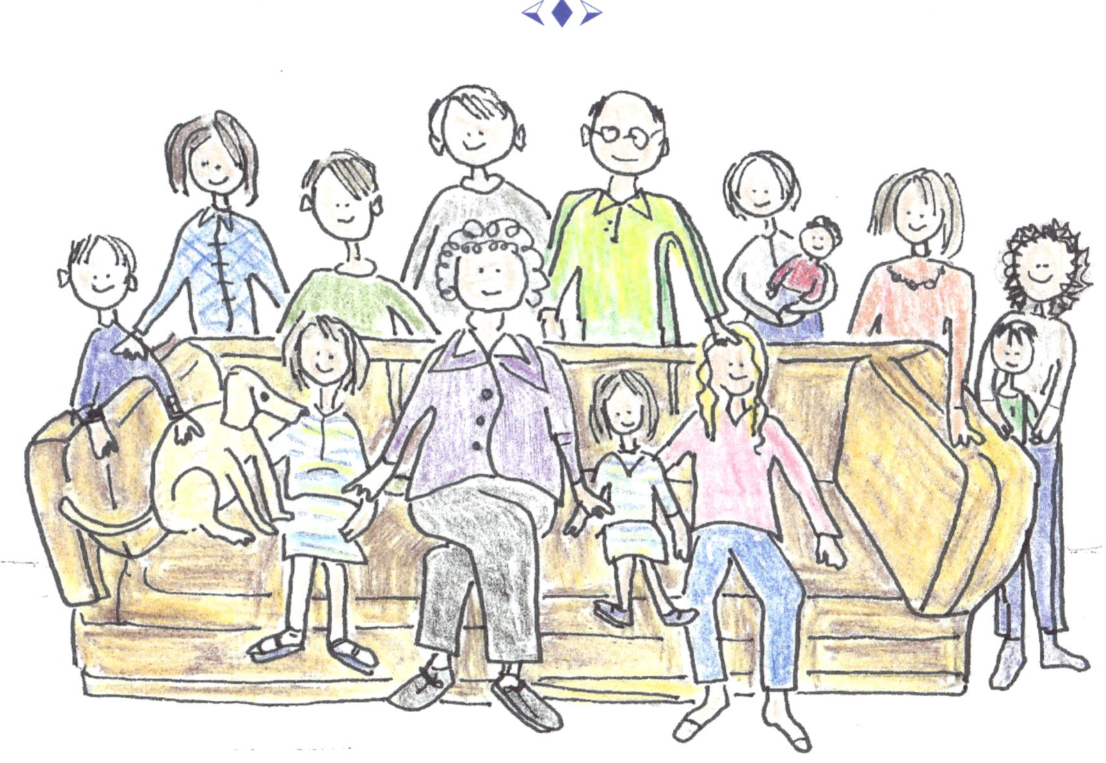

"It is nice to have your friends so close by, friends who are going through many of the same things you are. That is what keeps me going."

"The people here accept aging with grace. There is a kindness among the residents. We feel cared for. We feel safe. We have each other. And, we have each other's back."

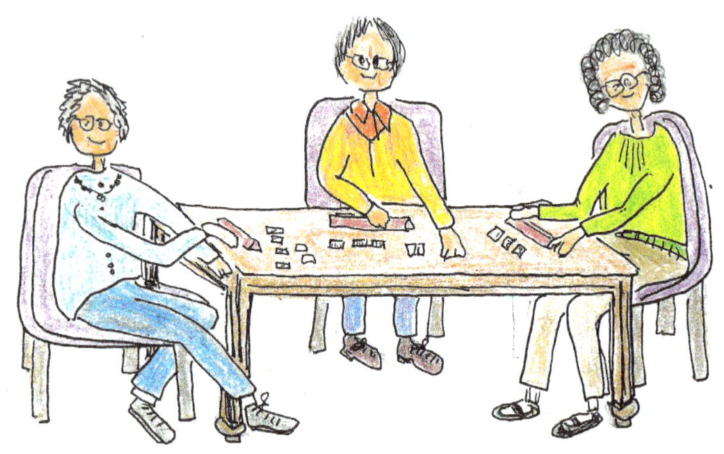

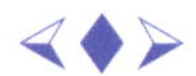

*"I have learned that I can live well even as I get older. I have had a wonderful life and it continues here where I have many more friends than I had before—it is the magic of the place. **My new old friends.**"*

9

THOUGHTS FOR OTHERS

This experiment in growing older seems to have worked for these women. And they do have thoughts to pass along to those junior to them—those in their late 70s and early 80s:

"If you stay in your home, you'll likely be lonely and aging can hurt more."

"At a place like this you can have independence from your kids but still have them in your life. Our children are thrilled we are in a senior living community, being taken care of—your children would be too."

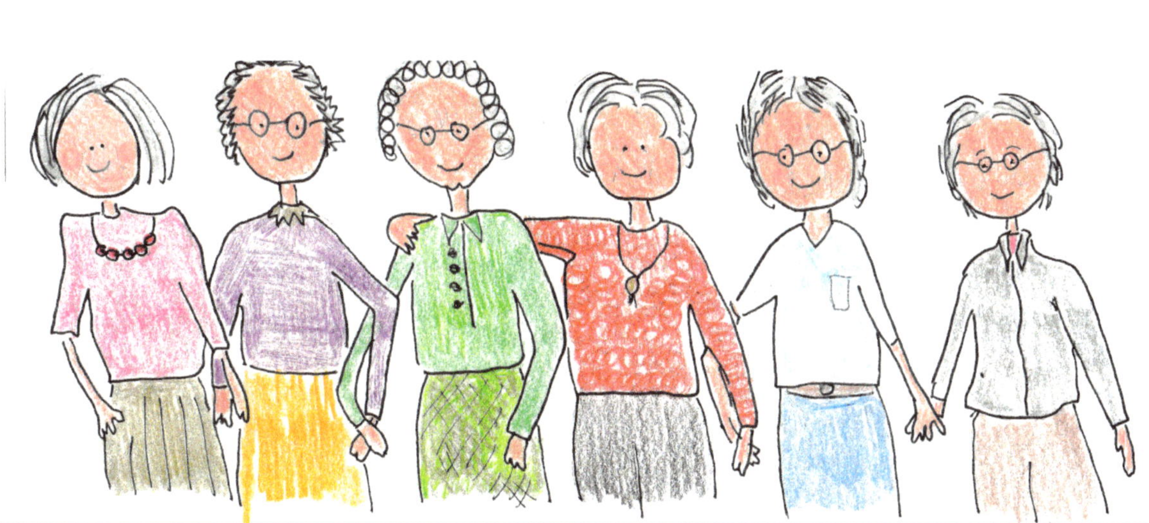

"Attitude is everything; if you are negative you will find the negative."

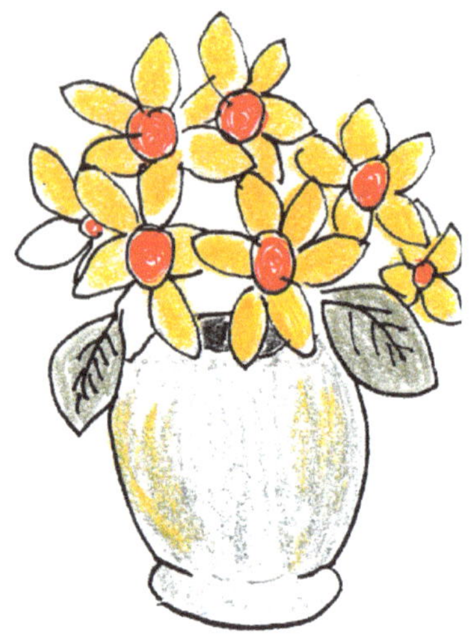

"Think of what you have, not what you don't have or have lost; and focus on what you can do now, not what you used to do."

"Try to keep your health, make sure you don't fall, and most importantly, do keep your friends close."

CONCLUSION: LIFE GOES ON

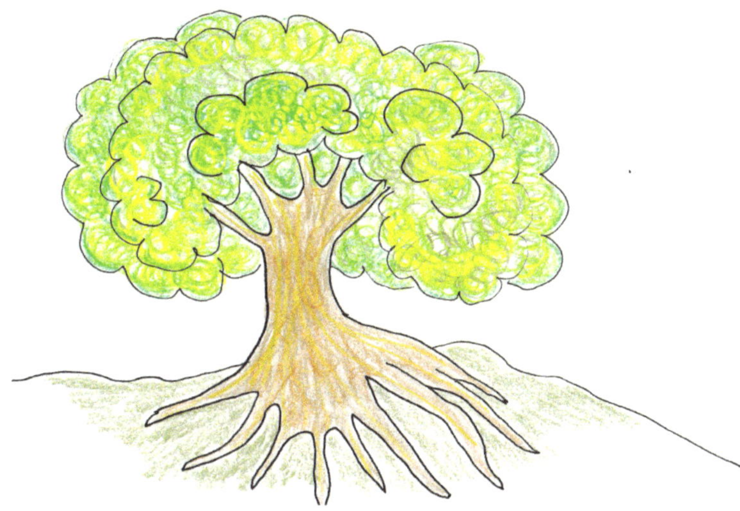

It was Monday evening, barely a month since Nancy passed away. Mimi sat at the dining room table with four friends. It would be the usual Monday group, but sitting in what would have been Nancy's chair was a woman who had just moved in to the Residence.

A new old friend.

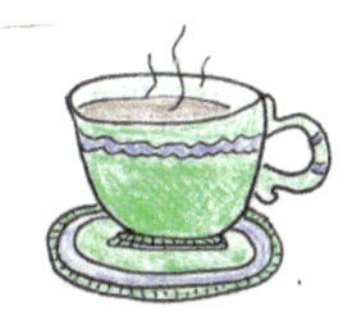

ACKNOWLEDGMENTS

I would like to thank the many women at the Residence with whom I have had the opportunity to talk, especially: Nancy, Julie, Liz, Sue, Vi, Eadie, Rei, Sissy, Lou Ann, Lois J, Muffy, Carol M, Celia, and Mimi. I deeply appreciate your thoughtful and honest discussion about life in your 90s.

And, a special nod to my editorial helpers—Julie, Amy, Kathe, Kaitlin, Pat, Vivian, Chris, and especially, Joann.

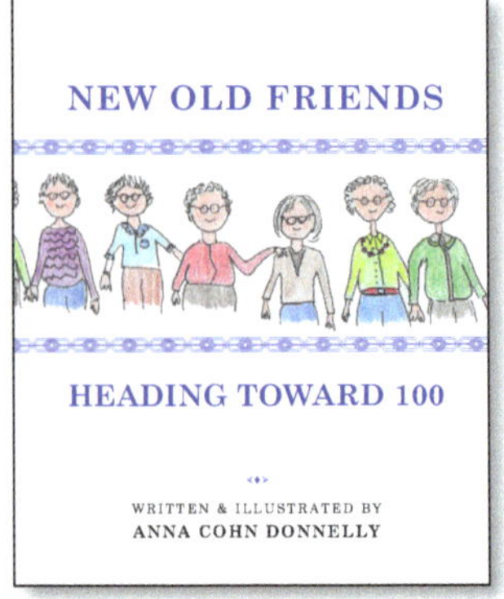

Books by author & illustrator, Anna Cohn Donnelly

Most would think of those in their 90s as ancient, with little to look forward to. **New Old Friends: Heading Toward 100**, a fully illustrated book, tells a different story from the point of view of fourteen women in their late eighties and nineties who live in a senior living community. All have had good lives and all have experienced great sorrow. They find that as they age, they actually gain a lot, most particularly, new old friends.

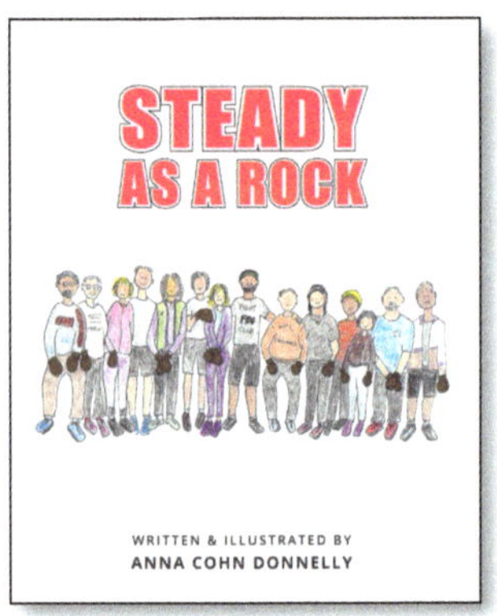

Steady as a Rock is a fully-illustrated inspiring story, told in the first person, of a group of senior citizens who find relief from the complications of Parkinson's and much more by regularly attending a boxing class entitled Rock Steady Boxing. By working out together, friendships abound and participants find they are no longer fighting alone the effects of the disease. The book documents the benefits of stepping out of your comfort zone.

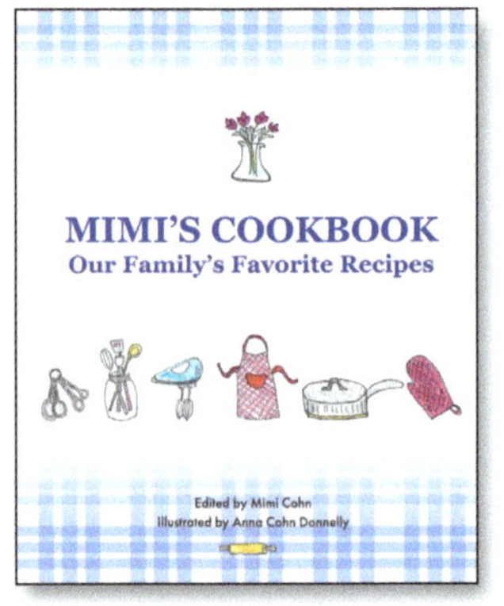

As she approached age 98, Mimi wanted to create something that would touch the whole family. Since we all love to eat and to cook, the idea of a cookbook that contained the family favorites made all the sense. **Mimi's Cookbook** is a collection of more than sixty odd favorites with illustrations.

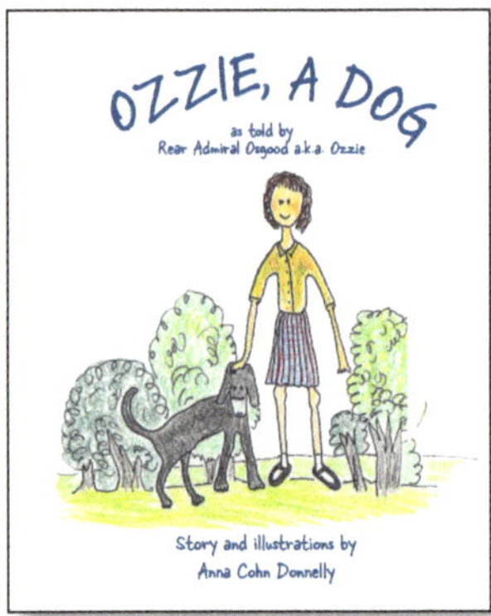

Ozzie, a black mutt, tells his story of being adopted by the large and active Cohn family from Jack's Dog Farm and finding adventure and love in his new home, particularly with the youngest child Julie who arrived after he did. This is a heartwarming tale, filled with illustrations, of life on four paws.

Books by author & illustrator, Anna Cohn Donnelly

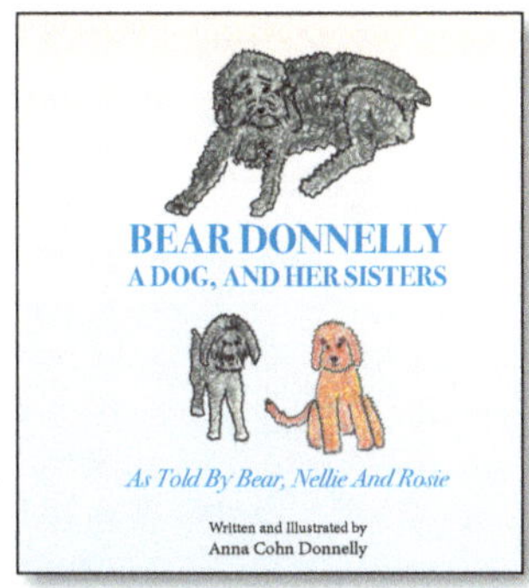

Bear Donnelly, A Dog, and Her Sisters, illustrated story told by Bear Donnelly, a 14 year old Bouvier de Flanders, of her life in the Donnelly household. Some of Bear's stories are happy ones, and some are not. Bear's younger sisters, Nellie and Rosie, also tell a bit about their lives.

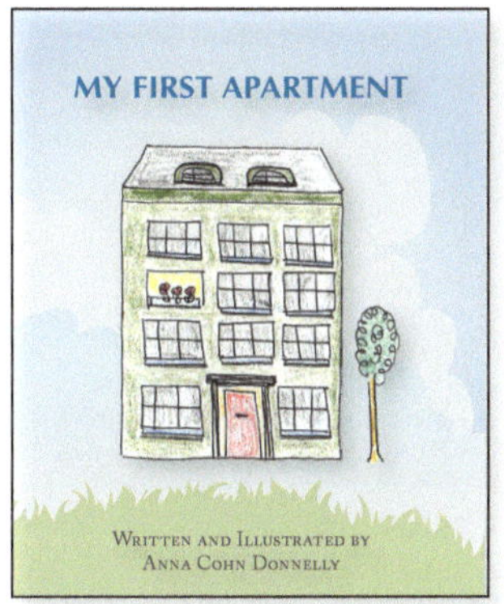

Having secured her first, real full time job, the youngest of four was leaving home to live downtown in an apartment with a school buddy. Rather than lecture her on the do's and do not's of living on her own, the author decided to cull advice from her older siblings and cousins and distill it in a short book. Written from the daughter's perspective, and fully-illustrated, ***My First Apartment*** offers guidance to those starting out on their own.

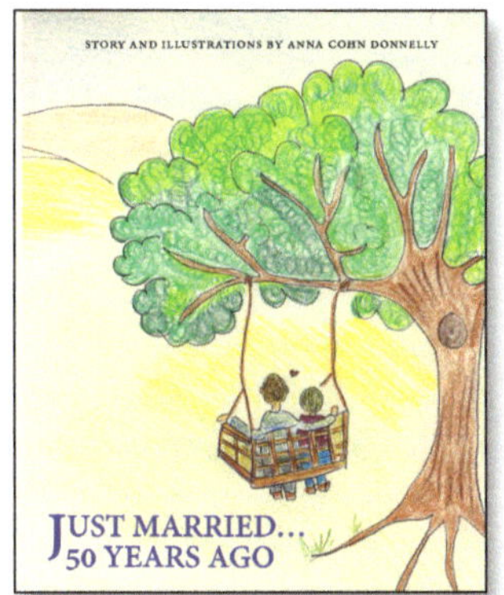

From the moment they met, David and Naida were in love. ***Just Married…50 Years Ago***, a fully-illustrated book, follows them through their first fifty years and documents the best that a marriage and committed partnership can offer.

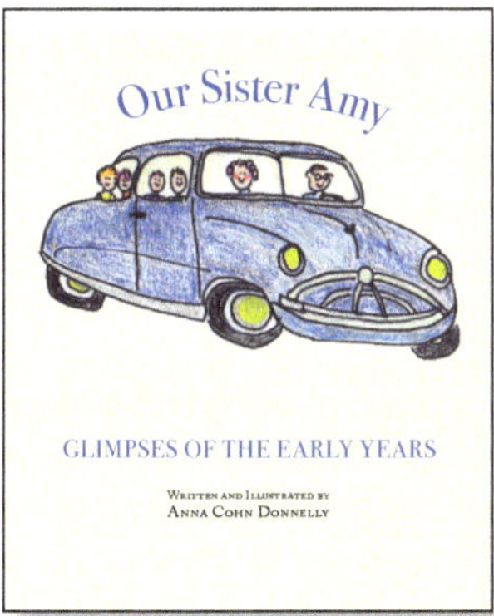

Amy was the fourth child of five, with two older brothers and an older sister and a younger one. She and her sister Anna, fourteen months her senior, had a profound impact on each other. ***Our Sister Amy***, fully-illustrated, provides glimpses into the early years of their lives together and characterizes just how precious the sister relationship can be, as they grow up, even as they compete and strive for independence.